About the NCCN Guidelines for Patients®

NCCN National Comprehensive Cancer Network®

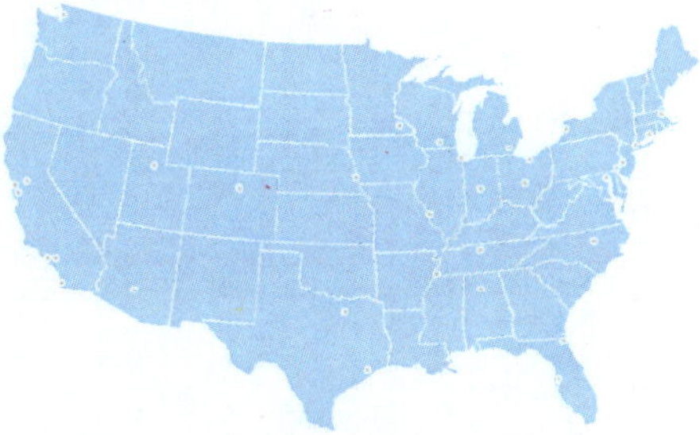

Did you know that top cancer centers across the United States work together to improve cancer care? This alliance of leading cancer centers is called the National Comprehensive Cancer Network® (NCCN®).

Cancer care is always changing. NCCN develops evidence-based cancer care recommendations used by health care providers worldwide. These frequently updated recommendations are the NCCN Clinical Practice Guidelines in Oncology (NCCN Guidelines®). The NCCN Guidelines for Patients plainly explain these expert recommendations for people with cancer and caregivers.

These NCCN Guidelines for Patients are based on the NCCN Clinical Practice Guidelines in Oncology (NCCN Guidelines®) for Pediatric Hodgkin Lymphoma, Version 2.2023 — March 9, 2023.

View the NCCN Guidelines for Patients free online
NCCN.org/patientguidelines

Find an NCCN Cancer Center near you
NCCN.org/cancercenters

Connect with us

Supporters

NCCN Guidelines for Patients are supported by funding from the NCCN Foundation®

NCCN Foundation gratefully acknowledges the following supporters for helping to make available these NCCN Guidelines for Patients: Seagen Inc.

NCCN independently adapts, updates, and hosts the NCCN Guidelines for Patients. Our corporate supporters do not participate in the development of the NCCN Guidelines for Patients and are not responsible for the content and recommendations contained therein.

To make a gift or learn more visit online or email

NCCNFoundation.org/donate

PatientGuidelines@NCCN.org

Contents

NCCN Foundation seeks to support the millions of patients and their families affected by a cancer diagnosis by funding and distributing NCCN Guidelines for Patients. NCCN Foundation is also committed to advancing cancer treatment by funding the nation's promising doctors at the center of innovation in cancer research. For more details and the full library of patient and caregiver resources, visit NCCN.org/patients.

National Comprehensive Cancer Network (NCCN) and NCCN Foundation
3025 Chemical Road, Suite 100, Plymouth Meeting, PA 19462 USA

1 Hodgkin lymphoma basics

With the right treatment, Hodgkin lymphoma can usually be cured. This is because the treatments for it have become safer and more effective. But late side effects of treatment can occur. Long-term follow-up is essential.

About Hodgkin lymphoma

Hodgkin lymphoma is an uncommon cancer of the lymph nodes and the lymphatic system. Most people are diagnosed between the ages of 15 to 30, or after age 55. It is the most common cancer in teenagers 15 to 19 years of age. It is less common in children between the ages of 5 and 14.

This guide provides treatment recommendations for children, adolescents, and young adults (up to age 39) diagnosed with Hodgkin lymphoma.

More information on Hodgkin lymphoma in older adults is available at NCCN.org/patientguidelines and on the NCCN Patient Guides for Cancer app.

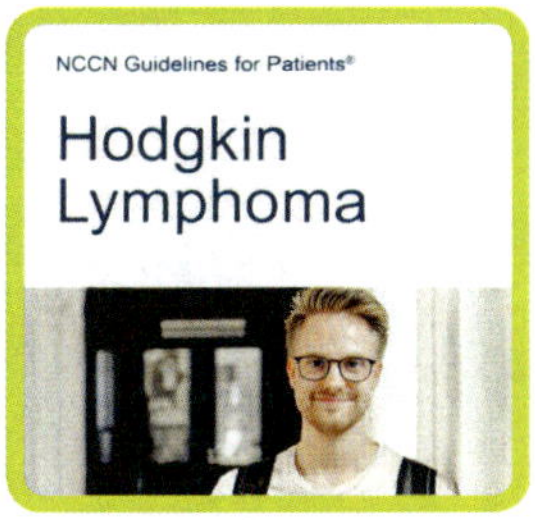

Key points

- ✓ Hodgkin lymphoma is a cancer of the immune system. It can often be cured with treatment.
- ✓ There are different types of Hodgkin lymphoma. The extent of the disease can vary from person to person.
- ✓ First steps involve scans and lab tests. The results will be used to develop a treatment plan.
- ✓ If available, participating in a clinical trial for treatment is highly encouraged if you are eligible.
- ✓ Chemotherapy is the most effective and widely used treatment for Hodgkin lymphoma.
- ✓ Radiation therapy may be given after chemotherapy.
- ✓ High-dose chemotherapy with stem cell rescue may be used to treat cancer that returns after treatment.
- ✓ Hodgkin lymphoma and its treatment can cause serious health problems many years later. Long-term follow-up care is essential.
- ✓ More detail on each of this steps is provided in this guide.

The lymphatic system

The lymphatic system helps the body fight infection and disease. It is part of the immune system. The tissues and organs of the lymphatic system are made mostly of white blood cells called lymphocytes. There are many other types of white blood cells, but lymphocytes are the most important for understanding Hodgkin lymphoma.

Lymph and lymphatic vessels

A super-highway of ducts, called lymphatic vessels, runs through the body. Much like how blood vessels transport blood, lymphatic vessels transport lymph. Lymph is a clear fluid made mostly of lymphocytes. It is also called lymphatic fluid.

Lymph nodes

While traveling throughout the body in lymphatic vessels, lymph passes through hundreds of small bean-shaped structures called lymph nodes. Lymph nodes filter out foreign particles, germs, and harmful cells, including cancer cells. Lymph nodes can't usually be seen or felt. Certain areas of the body contain more lymph nodes than others. The highest numbers of lymph nodes are found in the:

- Neck (cervical lymph nodes)
- Groin (inguinal lymph nodes)
- Armpits (axillary lymph nodes)

Spleen

The spleen is the largest organ of the lymphatic system. It is about 4 inches long and shaped like a fist. Like lymph nodes, the spleen contains lymphocytes that help the body fight infection and disease. The spleen also plays an important role in blood filtration and storage.

Bone marrow

Most bones have soft, spongy tissue in the center called bone marrow. This is where new blood cells, including some lymphocytes, are made. B lymphocytes (B cells), 1 of 2 main types of lymphocytes, are made in the bone marrow. The "B" in B cells stands for bone marrow.

Thymus

The thymus is a small organ in the upper chest. Here, early lymphocytes develop into T lymphocytes (T cells), the other main type of lymphocyte. The "T" in T cells stands for thymus.

The tonsils

Tonsils are small masses of lymph tissue found at the back of the throat. They help trap disease-causing germs that enter through your nose or mouth.

Lymphatic system

Hodgkin lymphoma spreads through lymphatic vessels from1 group of lymph nodes to the next. If left untreated, it will spread to tissue and organs outside the lymphatic system.

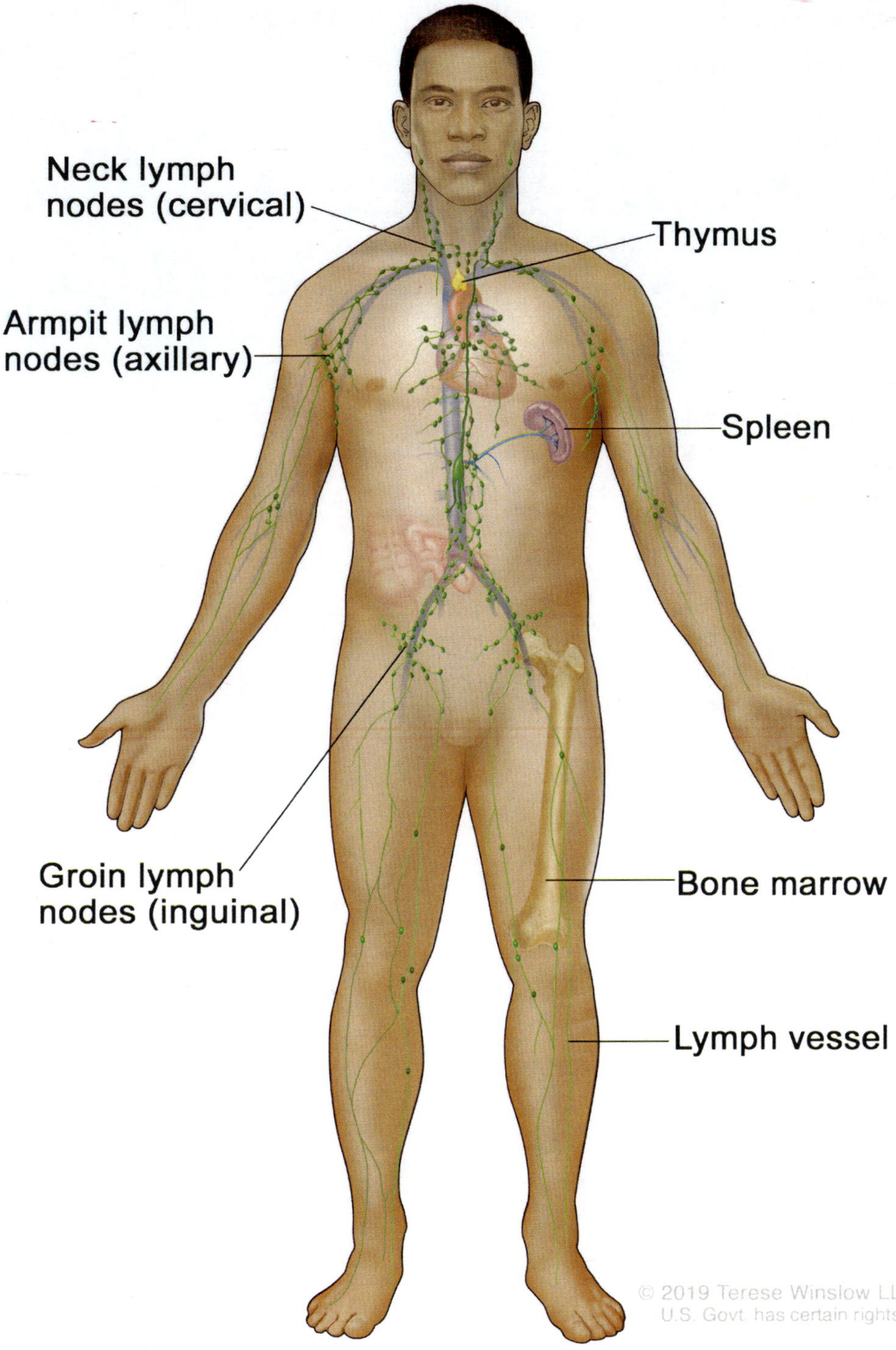

Types of Hodgkin lymphoma

CHL

Most people diagnosed with Hodgkin lymphoma have classic Hodgkin lymphoma (CHL). There are 4 types of CHL:

- Nodular sclerosis (most common)
- Mixed cellularity
- Lymphocyte-rich
- Lymphocyte-depleted (least common)

While they are all considered CHL, they look different under a microscope. They may also behave differently. For example, some types are more likely to cause symptoms than others. The CHL treatment information in this guide applies to all 4 subtypes.

NLPHL

Only about 1 in 20 people with Hodgkin lymphoma have nodular lymphocyte predominant Hodgkin lymphoma (NLPHL). This rare type is slow-growing. Over time, in rare cases, NLPHL can become an aggressive type of non-Hodgkin lymphoma called diffuse large B-cell lymphoma (DLBCL).

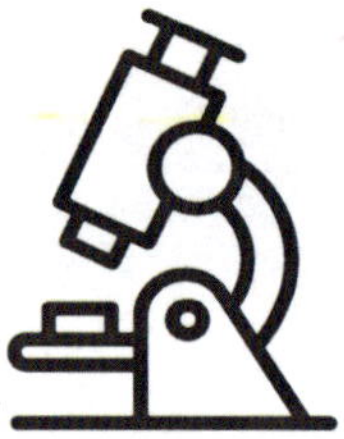

Doctors can tell if a suspected cancer is Hodgkin lymphoma by looking at one or more lymph nodes under a microscope. In CHL, abnormally large lymphocytes called Reed-Sternberg cells can be seen. Experts don't know why normal lymphocytes turn into Reed-Sternberg cells.

Non-Hodgkin lymphomas are a large and varied group of lymphomas. They do not have the distinctive Reed-Sternberg cells seen in Hodgkin lymphoma. This book does not discuss treatment of non-Hodgkin lymphomas.

Clinical trials

A clinical trial is a type of medical research study. After being developed and tested in a laboratory, potential new ways of fighting cancer need to be studied in people. If found to be safe and effective in a clinical trial, a drug, device, or treatment approach may be approved by the U.S. Food and Drug Administration (FDA).

Everyone with cancer should carefully consider all of the treatment options available for their cancer type, including standard treatments and clinical trials. Talk to your doctor about whether a clinical trial may make sense for you.

Phases

Most cancer clinical trials focus on treatment. Treatment trials are done in phases.

- **Phase 1** trials study the dose, safety, and side effects of an investigational drug or treatment approach. They also look for early signs that the drug or approach is helpful.
- **Phase 2** trials study how well the drug or approach works against a specific type of cancer.
- **Phase 3** trials test the drug or approach against a standard treatment. If the results are good, it may be approved by the FDA.
- **Phase 4** trials study the long-term safety and benefit of an FDA-approved treatment.

Who can enroll?

Every clinical trial has rules for joining, called eligibility criteria. The rules may be about age, cancer type and stage, treatment history, or general health. These requirements ensure that participants are alike in specific ways and that the trial is as safe as possible for the participants.

Finding a clinical trial

In the United States

NCCN Cancer Centers
NCCN.org/cancercenters

The National Cancer Institute (NCI)
cancer.gov/about-cancer/treatment/clinical-trials/search

Worldwide

The U.S. National Library of Medicine (NLM)
clinicaltrials.gov

Need help finding a clinical trial?

NCI's Cancer Information Service (CIS)
1.800.4.CANCER (1.800.422.6237)
cancer.gov/contact

Informed consent

Clinical trials are managed by a group of experts called a research team. The research team will review the study with you in detail, including its purpose and the risks and benefits of participating. All of this information is also provided in an informed consent form. Read the form carefully and ask questions before signing it. Take time to discuss it with family, friends, or others you trust. Keep in mind that you can leave and seek treatment outside of the clinical trial at any time.

Start the conversation

Don't wait for your doctor to bring up clinical trials. Start the conversation and learn about all of your treatment options. If you find a study that you may be eligible for, ask your treatment team if you meet the requirements. If you have already started standard treatment, you may not be eligible for certain clinical trials. Try not to be discouraged if you cannot join. New clinical trials are always becoming available.

Frequently asked questions

There are many myths and misconceptions surrounding clinical trials. The possible benefits and risks are not well understood by many with cancer.

Will I get a placebo?
Placebos (inactive versions of real medicines) are almost never used alone in cancer clinical trials. It is common to receive either a placebo with a standard treatment or a new drug with a standard treatment. You will be informed, verbally and in writing, if a placebo is part of a clinical trial before you enroll.

Are clinical trials free?
There is no fee to enroll in a clinical trial. The study sponsor pays for research-related costs, including the study drug. You may, however, have costs indirectly related to the trial, such as the cost of transportation or child care due to extra appointments. During the trial, you will continue to receive standard cancer care. This care is billed to—and often covered by—insurance. You are responsible for copays and any costs for this care that are not covered by your insurance.

Key points

Basics

- Hodgkin lymphoma is an uncommon cancer of the lymph nodes and the lymphatic system.
- Most people are diagnosed between the ages of 15 to 30, or after age 55.
- It is the most common cancer in teens 15 to 19 years of age.
- Most young people with Hodgkin lymphoma are cured with chemotherapy. Radiation therapy may also be given.

Types of Hodgkin lymphoma

- Most people diagnosed with Hodgkin lymphoma have classic Hodgkin lymphoma (CHL).
- Types of CHL include nodular sclerosis, mixed cellularity, lymphocyte-rich, and lymphocyte-depleted.
- Nodular lymphocyte-predominant Hodgkin lymphoma (NLPHL) is a rare type of Hodgkin lymphoma.

Clinical trials

- Treatment for Hodgkin lymphoma has steadily improved because of clinical trials.
- Receiving treatment as part of a clinical trial is recommended for this uncommon cancer.
- Ask your care team if a trial is available and if you are eligible to participate.

2

Testing for Hodgkin lymphoma

This chapter describes the tests used to diagnose and stage Hodgkin lymphoma. Other testing and care you may have before treatment is explained.

Physical exam

Your doctor will review your health history and perform a physical exam. Normally, lymph nodes can't be seen or felt. But Hodgkin lymphoma can cause them to get bigger than normal. Using their hands, your doctor will feel the areas of the body where there are the most lymph nodes. This includes the neck, armpits, and groin. In addition to these areas, expect your doctor to feel your spleen and liver.

Symptoms

Hodgkin lymphoma can cause symptoms. There are 3 in particular that your doctor should be aware of, if you have them. These are called "B" symptoms. They include:

- Unexplained fevers (above 100.4 degrees Fahrenheit)
- Heavy, drenching night sweats
- Noticeable weight loss without trying to lose weight

The symptoms listed below may also be related to Hodgkin lymphoma.

- Itchy skin
- Extreme tiredness
- A bad reaction to alcohol

B symptoms

Fever

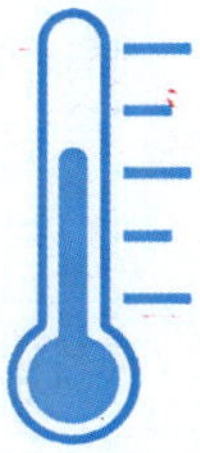

Heavy night sweats

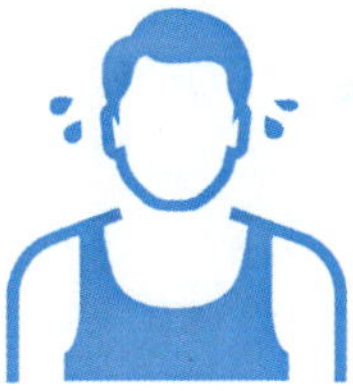

Unexplained weight loss

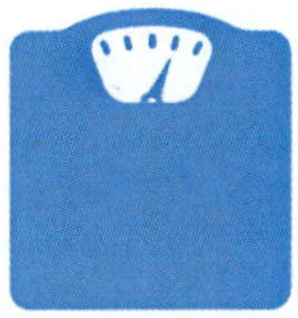

Lymph node biopsy

A lymph node biopsy is needed to diagnose Hodgkin lymphoma. Either an excisional or incisional biopsy is preferred. In an excisional biopsy, one or more whole lymph nodes are removed and tested. In an incisional or "open" biopsy, a small amount of lymph node tissue is removed through a cut in the skin. These procedures are usually done under general anesthesia.

While these types are preferred, a core needle biopsy is sometimes performed. This type involves the use of a wide needle to remove a sample of tissue from a lymph node. The lymph node itself is not removed. This can often be done with local anesthesia or deep sedation.

Another type of biopsy called a fine-needle aspiration (FNA) should not be used alone to diagnose Hodgkin lymphoma. In an FNA, a thin needle is used to remove a sample of tissue from a lymph node. This is typically done with a local anesthetic.

Testing the removed node(s)

The removed lymph nodes are examined under a microscope to look for the abnormally large Reed-Sternberg cells that are seen in classic Hodgkin lymphoma (CHL).

The tissue is also tested using a process called immunohistochemistry. Using a microscope, this test looks for proteins on the surface of cells. A diagnosis can be made based on the proteins that can be seen (and not seen). For example, in CHL, proteins called CD15 and CD30 can usually be seen on the surface of Reed-Sternberg cells, while CD3 and CD45 usually cannot.

In the case of nodular lymphocyte-predominant Hodgkin lymphoma (NLPHL), a surface protein called CD20 can usually be seen but CD15 and CD30 usually cannot.

Blood tests

The blood tests typically done as part of testing for Hodgkin lymphoma are described below.

A complete blood count (CBC) measures the number of red blood cells, white blood cells, and platelets in a sample of blood.

An erythrocyte sedimentation rate (ESR) test measures how quickly red blood cells settle at the bottom of a test tube that contains a blood sample. A higher-than-normal ESR may be a sign of inflammation, infection, cancer, or other diseases.

C-reactive protein (CRP) is a protein made by the liver when there is inflammation in the body. A high level of CRP can be a sign of infection, cancer, rheumatoid arthritis, lupus, or heart problems.

A comprehensive metabolic panel (CMP) is a group of more than 10 blood tests. It provides information about the health of the kidneys, liver, and other organs and tissues. It also gives information on your blood sugar, calcium, and electrolytes.

Before starting treatment, those who are able to become pregnant should have a pregnancy test. Testing for human immunodeficiency virus (HIV) and for hepatitis B and C is encouraged, especially if your doctor thinks you may be at risk for these diseases.

Testing for immune system problems (immunodeficiency) may be ordered for children under the age of 5. It is often also considered for those with:

- Repeat infections, or
- Non-typical signs or symptoms, or
- A personal or family history of immunodeficiency.

Imaging

PET

Positron emission tomography (PET) scans use a small amount of radioactive glucose (sugar), called a radiotracer. Fluorodeoxyglucose (FDG) is most often used. The tracer gives off a small amount of energy that is detected by the scanner. Areas with cancer appear brighter ("hotter") because cancer cells use sugar more quickly than normal cells.

A 5-point system, called the Deauville criteria, is used to rate how much of the tracer is absorbed by areas with cancer compared to how much is absorbed by the liver and the mediastinum (the area between the lungs).

A Deauville score of 1 or 2 means that there are no cancerous areas of concern. A score of 4 or 5 generally means that there are cancerous areas of concern. A score of 3 can be considered good or bad, depending on the situation.

FDG-PET scans are used to determine the cancer stage and to see how well treatment is working. It is common to have more than one FDG-PET scan during the course of treatment. FDG-PET is often combined with either computed tomography or magnetic resonance imaging.

CT and MRI

Computed tomography (CT) and magnetic resonance imaging (MRI) are other important imaging tests used for Hodgkin lymphoma. As part of initial testing, it is common to have a CT scan of the area from the neck to the groin.

Imaging for Hodgkin lymphoma

In addition to FDG-PET scans, CT and MRI are important imaging tests used for Hodgkin lymphoma. Contrast is often given for CT and MRI scans.

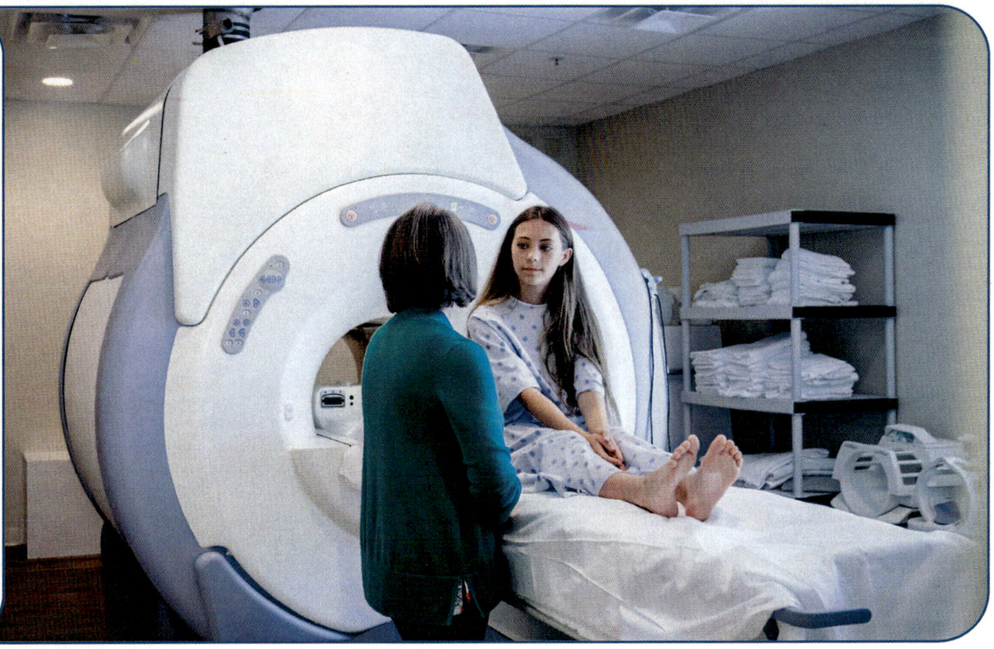

Or you may have a combination of a CT scan and an MRI of separate areas of your body. Depending on the type of PET/CT or PET/MRI obtained in your workup, you may not need separate CT and MRI scans.

CT takes many pictures of a body part from different angles using x-rays. A computer combines the x-rays to make detailed pictures.

MRI uses radio waves and powerful magnets to take pictures of areas inside the body. It does not use radiation. Because of the very strong magnets used in the MRI machine, tell the technician if you have any metal in your body.

Contrast

Contrast is a substance put into the body that makes imaging pictures clearer. It is often used for CT and MRI scans. The contrast is put into the bloodstream through a vein and may also be given as a drink. Tell your care team if you have had problems with contrast in the past. Allergic reactions, such as throat swelling and hives, are possible. You will be asked a series of questions to make sure you are not allergic to the contrast.

Heart and lung tests

Some cancer treatments can damage the heart and lungs. In order to plan treatment, your doctors will test how well your heart and lungs work.

Echocardiogram

An echocardiogram uses sound waves to see how well the heart is working. A technician called a cardiac sonographer performs this test. The technician slides a wand with gel on its tip across your chest. They are able to view your beating heart on a screen. The pictures are recorded for future viewing.

If chemotherapy containing an anthracycline is planned, an echocardiogram is recommended. Doxorubicin is an anthracycline used in some chemotherapy regimens used to treat Hodgkin lymphoma.

Electrocardiogram

An electrocardiogram (ECG or EKG) may be helpful in some cases. This test shows electrical changes in the heart. It reveals information about heart rate and rhythm. For this test, small patches are placed on the chest to track the heartbeat.

Lung function tests

Bleomycin is a chemotherapy medicine sometimes used (with other medicines) to treat Hodgkin lymphoma in young people. Bleomycin can damage the lungs. If treatment that includes bleomycin is being considered, lung function tests are recommended. The 3 most common lung function tests are described below.

- **Spirometry measures** the amount of air the lungs can hold, and how fast you can empty the air out of your lungs.
- **A gas diffusion test** involves breathing in a harmless gas and measuring how much of it you breathe out. It tells how much oxygen travels from your lungs into your blood.
- **Body plethysmograph** involves sitting in a small room and breathing into a tube. This test measures how much air your lungs can hold and how much air is left in your lungs after you exhale.

Other testing and care

Fertility and pregnancy

Most young people will have chemotherapy with a regimen that is unlikely to cause infertility. But if you want the option of having children after treatment or are unsure, tell your care team. There are ways to preserve your fertility. The most common methods are described next.

Sperm banking stores semen for later use by freezing it in liquid nitrogen. The medical term for this is semen cryopreservation.

Like sperm, unfertilized eggs can be removed, frozen, and stored for later use. This is called egg freezing or oocyte cryopreservation.

Ovarian tissue banking involves removing part or all of an ovary and freezing the part that contains the eggs. The frozen tissue containing the eggs can later be unfrozen and put back in the body.

More information on fertility preservation in adolescents and young adults is available at NCCN.org/patientguidelines and on the NCCN Patient Guides for Cancer app.

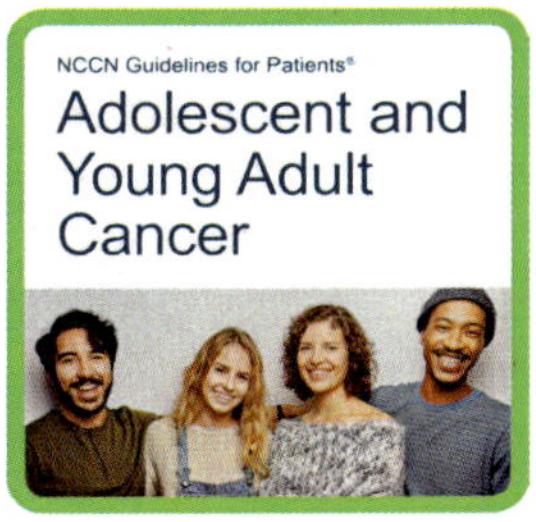

Before starting treatment, testing for pregnancy is recommended for anyone with Hodgkin lymphoma who could become pregnant.

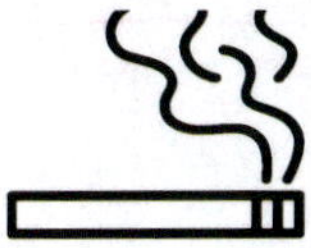

If you smoke or vape, seek help to quit

If you smoke or vape, it's important to quit. Smoking can limit how well cancer treatment works. Smoking and vaping can also increase the risk of lung problems during and after chemotherapy. It also increases your chances of developing other cancers.

Nicotine is the chemical in tobacco that makes you want to keep smoking. Nicotine withdrawal is challenging for most people who smoke. The stress of having cancer may make it even harder to quit. If you smoke, ask your doctor about counseling and medicines to help you quit.

For online support, try these websites:

- SmokeFree.gov
- BeTobaccoFree.gov
- CDC.gov/tobacco

Vaccines

The influenza vaccine (the "flu shot") is recommended for everyone with Hodgkin lymphoma, even during treatment.

If treating the spleen with radiation therapy is planned, certain vaccines are recommended before or after treatment. These include the vaccines for pneumonia, meningitis, and Haemophilus influenzae type B ("Hib" or "H-flu"). Despite its name, H-flu does not cause the common flu. It is a bacteria that can cause pneumonia and other serious infections, such as meningitis.

The COVID-19 vaccine can affect the appearance of your lymph nodes on FDG-PET, CT, and MRI scans. The lymph nodes may appear "hotter" on PET and larger on CT and MRI, usually on the side you received the vaccine. It is important to tell your doctors and imaging technicians that you have received this vaccine.

Bone marrow biopsy

In general, bone marrow biopsies are no longer included in the testing for Hodgkin lymphoma. But if you have lower-than-normal numbers of blood cells on complete blood count (CBC) and a PET scan doesn't suggest there is cancer in the bone marrow, a bone marrow biopsy may be needed.

Key points

Physical exam

- Your doctor will perform a full physical exam including examining your neck, armpits, and groin. These areas have the most lymph nodes.
- "B" symptoms include unexplained fevers (not caused by infection), heavy night sweats, and weight loss.

Biopsy

- A lymph node biopsy is needed to diagnose Hodgkin lymphoma. Either an excisional or incisional biopsy is preferred.

Imaging

- FDG-PET scans are used to determine the cancer stage and to see how well treatment is working. FDG-PET is often combined with either CT or MRI.

Heart and lung testing

- If chemotherapy with an anthracycline (such as doxorubicin) is planned, an echocardiogram is recommended.
- An electrocardiogram (ECG or EKG) can be helpful in some cases.
- If treatment that includes bleomycin is being considered, lung function tests are recommended.

Other testing and care

- If you smoke or vape, it is important to quit. Ask your care team for help.
- Most young people receive chemotherapy that is unlikely to cause infertility. If fertility preservation is needed, ask your care team about your options.

3

Staging

Before starting treatment, it is important to determine how far the cancer has spread. This process is called staging.

Overview and stages

The results of the physical exam and imaging tests are used to assign the stage.

Hodgkin lymphoma usually starts in the upper body, often in lymph nodes in the neck, chest, or armpits. The diaphragm is a thin muscle below the lungs and heart. It can be thought of as a dividing line between the chest and the abdomen. Hodgkin lymphoma is staged in part depending on whether cancer has spread to lymph nodes or other areas below the diaphragm.

There are 4 stages: I (1), II (2), III (3), and IV (4). One or more of the following letters may accompany the stage. They provide further information about the cancer.

- A – The cancer is asymptomatic (not causing "B" symptoms).
- B – There are B symptoms, such as fevers, night sweats, and weight loss.
- X –The lymph nodes with cancer are bulky (large).
- E – Cancer cells have invaded the non-lymphatic tissue next to or surrounding the lymph nodes. This is called an extralymphatic lesion or “e-lesion.”

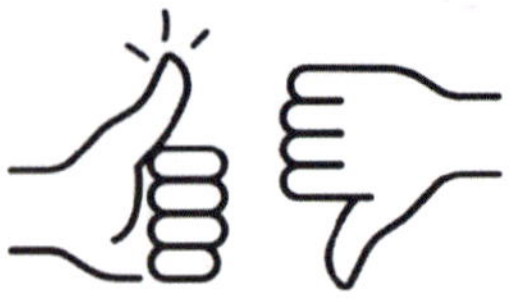

Let us know what you think!

Please take a moment to complete an online survey about the NCCN Guidelines for Patients.

NCCN.org/patients/response

Stage I

There is cancer in 1 group of lymph nodes, usually in the neck.

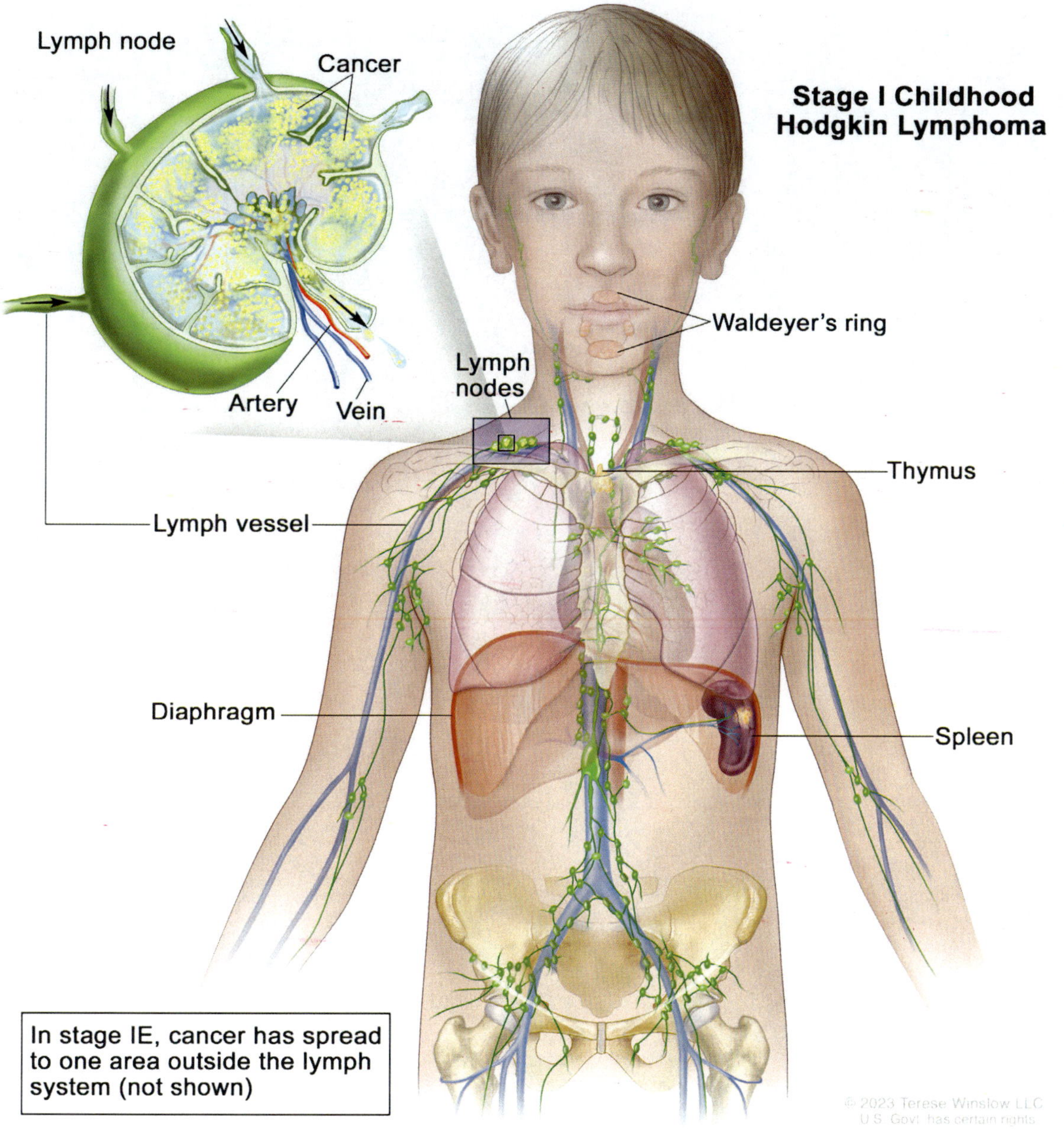

Stage 2

There is cancer in 2 or more groups of lymph nodes on the same side of the diaphragm (either above or below). In stage 2E (not shown), cancer cells have grown beyond lymph nodes into surrounding, non-lymphatic tissue.

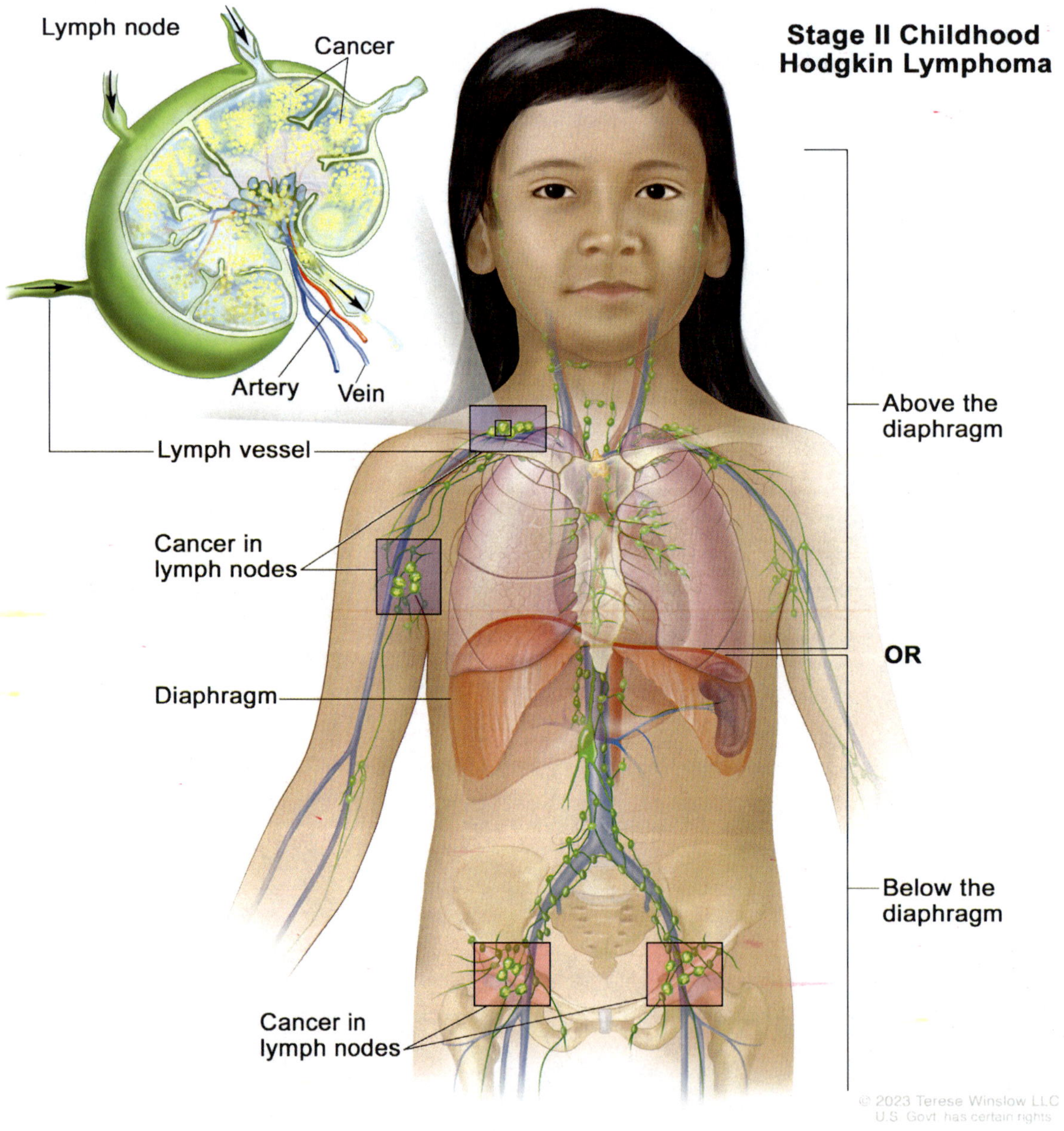

Stage 3

There is cancer in lymph nodes on both sides of the diaphragm.

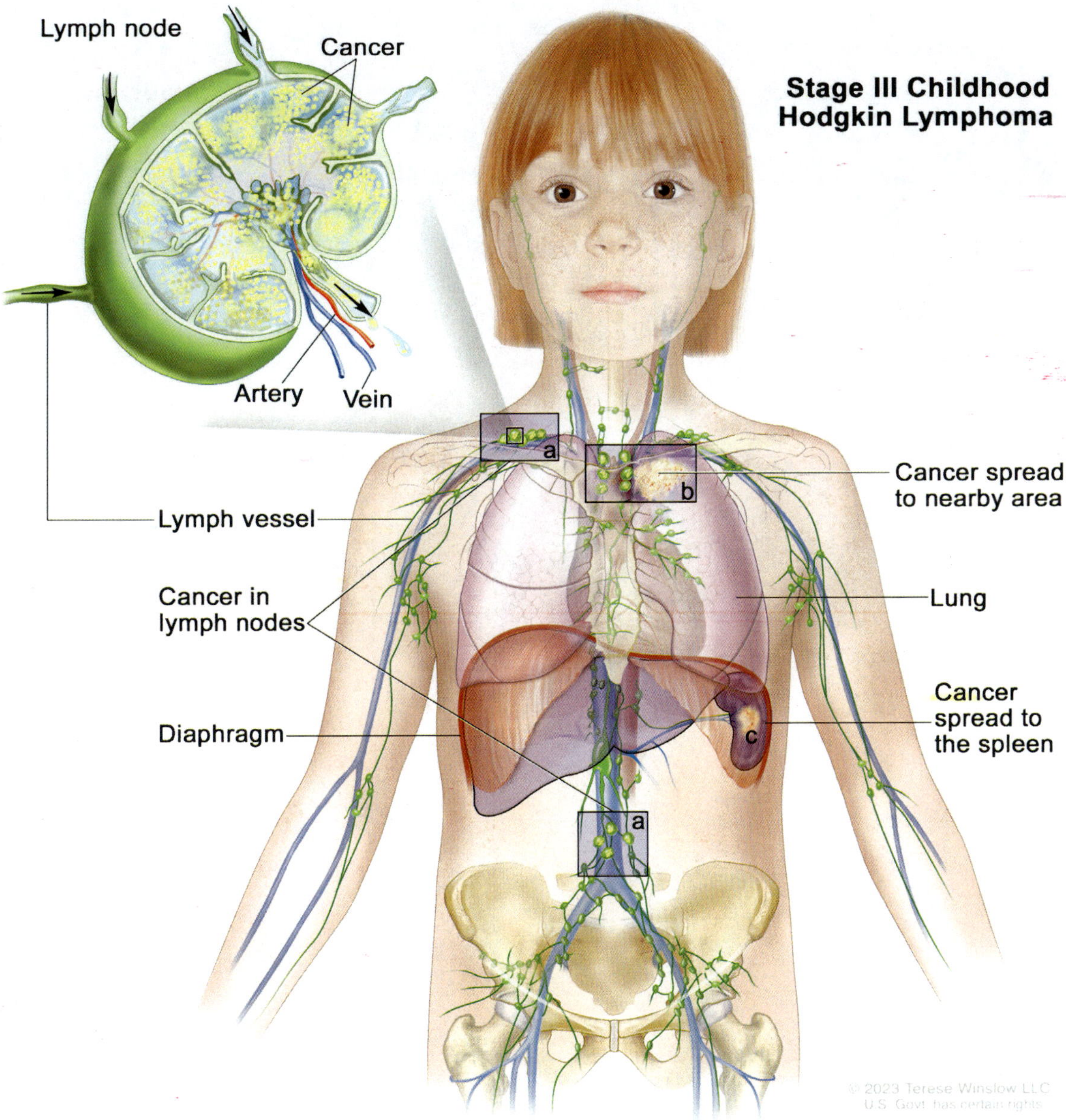

Stage 4

Cancer has spread to bone marrow or to organs outside of the lymphatic system, such as the lungs or liver.

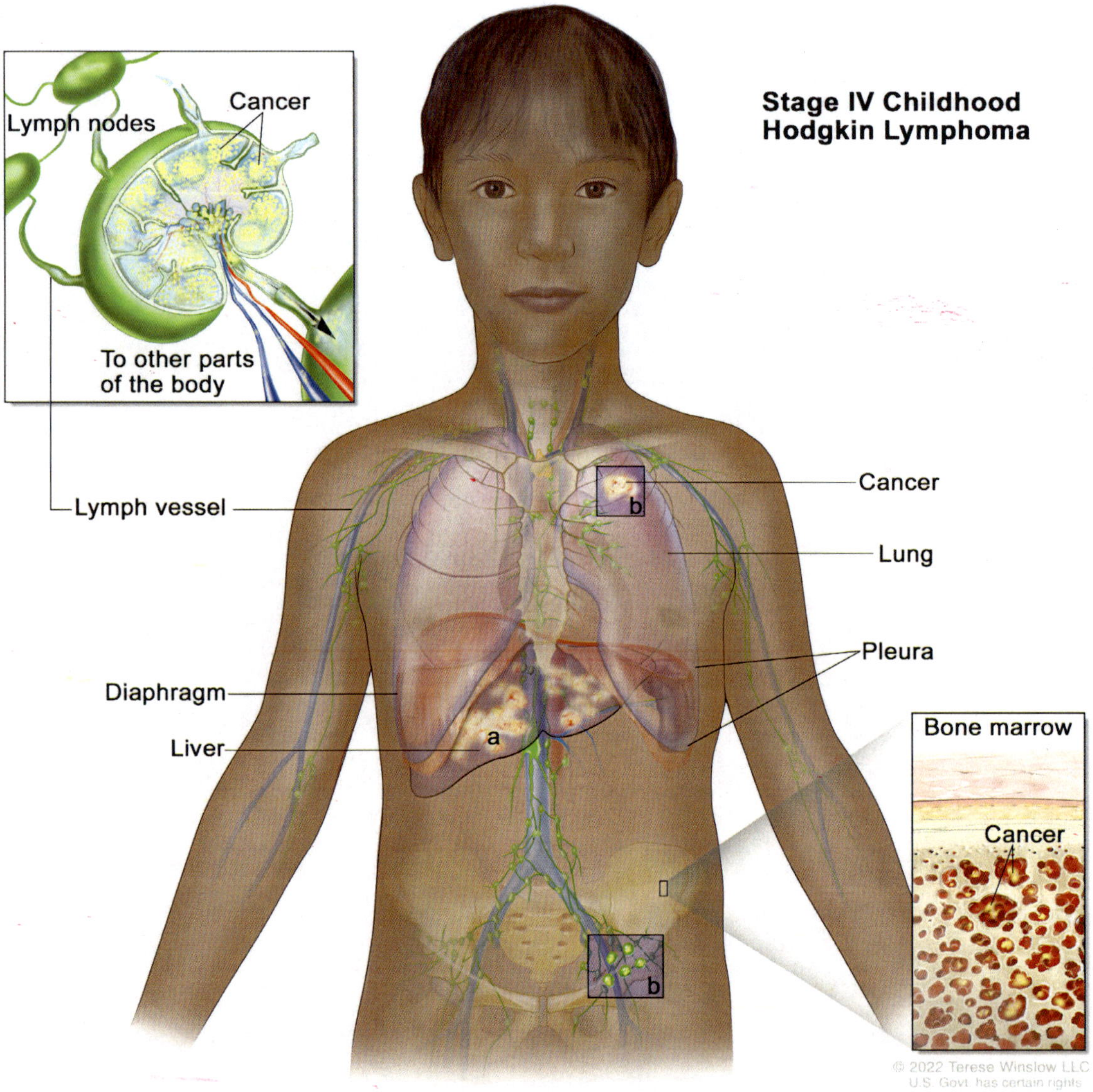

Key points

- The cancer stage describes the extent of cancer in the body.
- The physical exam and imaging results are used to determine the stage.
- Hodgkin lymphoma usually starts in lymph nodes in the neck, chest, or armpits.
- The cancer is staged based in part on whether it has spread to lymph nodes or other areas above or below the diaphragm.
- There are 4 stages: I (1), II (2), III (3), and IV (4).
- One or more letters providing extra information may accompany the stage.

The power of support

Seek out support groups at your treatment center, through social media, or from the resources listed in the back of this book. Look to friends, relatives, neighbors, and co-workers for social support. Many people find support groups helpful even after treatment is over. It can help with anxiety about cancer returning (recurrence).

4

Treatment for classic Hodgkin lymphoma (CHL)

Treatment for CHL starts with chemotherapy. Options for chemotherapy are based on the risk level of the cancer. Radiation therapy may follow chemotherapy.

Features seen in one person with Hodgkin lymphoma may not be seen in another with the same diagnosis. Over time, doctors have found that cancers with certain features need more intensive treatment. These features include:

- B symptoms (fevers, night sweats, weight loss)
- Bulky (large) lymph nodes with cancer
- Cancer outside of lymph nodes (higher stage cancer)
- Cancer in more than 1 group of lymph nodes
- Blood tests signaling inflammation

Treatment is based on whether the cancer has any of the above features. There are 3 risk groups: low, medium, and high. Tailoring the amount of chemotherapy according to risk group helps those with higher-stage cancer do just as well as those with lower-stage cancer.

At this time, there isn't one system that all doctors use to assign the cancer a risk group. And, risk grouping is always changing as new data become available. Ask your doctor which risk group applies to your cancer.

Regardless of risk level, seeking treatment within a clinical trial is strongly encouraged. Ask your care team if a trial is available and if you are eligible to participate.

Treatments

Chemotherapy

Chemotherapy is the most effective and widely used treatment for Hodgkin lymphoma. It is a type of systemic therapy. Systemic therapy is the use of medicine to kill cancer cells.

Most chemotherapies are liquids that are slowly injected into a vein. This process is called infusion. The drugs travel in the bloodstream to treat cancer throughout the body. Chemotherapy harms healthy cells in addition to cancer cells. This is why it can cause harsh side effects.

Chemotherapy is given in cycles of treatment days followed by days of rest. This allows the body to recover between cycles. Cycles vary in length depending on which drugs are used.

Brentuximab vedotin

Initial chemotherapy for **high-risk** CHL may include brentuximab vedotin (Adcetris). This antibody therapy combines 2 drugs in one. The antibody component (brentuximab) finds and attaches to cancer cells that have the CD30 protein on their surface, such as abnormally large Reed-Sternberg cells seen in CHL. Once attached, a chemotherapy drug is released into the cancer cell. By targeting only cells with CD30 receptors, fewer normal cells are harmed.

Radiation therapy

Radiation therapy may be given after initial chemotherapy for Hodgkin lymphoma. Using high-energy x-rays (photons), electrons, or protons, radiation therapy kills existing cancer cells or stops new cancer cells from being made.

If radiation therapy is needed, **involved-site radiation therapy (ISRT)** is often recommended. This type of external radiation therapy targets the lymph nodes in which the cancer started and nearby areas of cancer.

A simulation session will be performed before treatment with radiation therapy starts. Pictures of the tumor will be taken, usually using a CT scan in the radiation treatment position. The pictures are used to determine the details of your treatment. You may be asked to hold your breath during the simulation scan or treatment to keep your heart and lungs from moving.

During treatment, you will lie on a table in the same position as done for simulation. A mesh mask, body mold, or other devices may be used to keep you from moving. You will be alone while the therapists operate the machine from a nearby control room.

Proton therapy

Proton therapy is a newer type of particle-based radiation therapy. It may reduce late side effects caused by treatment with radiation, such as heart disease and second cancers. This is especially true for younger people with lymphoma in the area between the lungs. If treatment with radiation therapy is planned, young people with Hodgkin lymphoma or their caregivers are encouraged to ask if proton therapy is right for them.

Radiation therapy

Radiation therapy may be given after chemotherapy to treat Hodgkin lymphoma. A type of external radiation therapy called involved-site radiation therapy (ISRT) targets the lymph nodes where the cancer started and nearby areas of cancer.

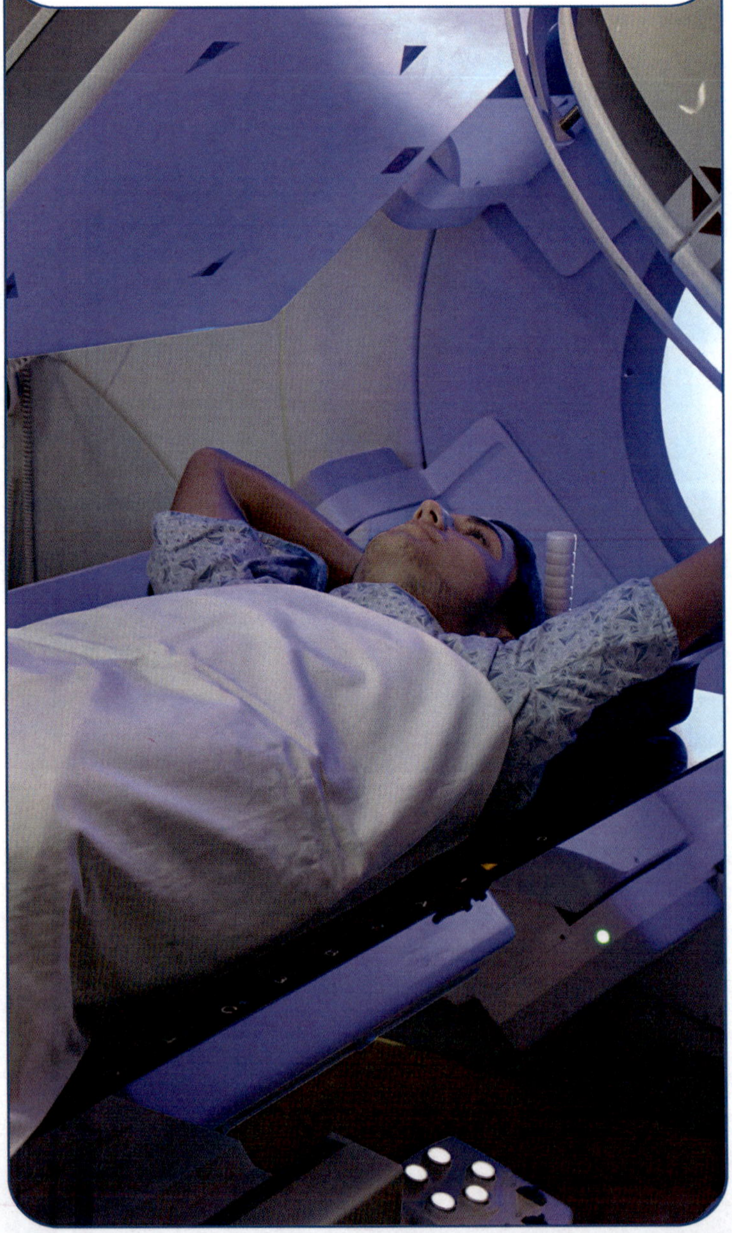

Low-risk CHL

Low-risk CHL includes non-bulky stage 1A and 2A cancers, and some stage 1B cancers. The cancer is contained within the nodes. When cancer cells grow beyond a lymph node into nearby non-lymphatic tissue, it is called an extralymphatic lesion or e-lesion. To be considered low-risk CHL, the cancer must not be bulky or have e-lesions.

Preferred treatment options

If a clinical trial is not available or otherwise not an option, chemotherapy with the OEPA regimen is preferred. The medicines included in this regimen are listed in **Guide 1** on page 32.

Treatment involves 2 cycles of OEPA. When complete, you will have a PET scan to see how well the treatment worked. The cancer will be designated as being either fast or slow to respond. If the cancer is designated as slow to respond, radiation therapy is recommended after chemotherapy.

If the response to chemotherapy is good, no further treatment is needed.

Other recommended options

For a small number of young people with CHL, the ABVD regimen may be considered. This regimen is usually used for adults. It is more toxic than regimens typically recommended for young people. It also has lower rates of success.

Less commonly used

If the cancer is the mixed cellularity subtype of CHL, 3 cycles of the AVPC regimen is recommended. If the response is good, no further treatment is needed. If the cancer does not improve enough with chemotherapy, radiation therapy is recommended.

Side effects

Managing side effects is a shared effort between you and your care team. It is important to speak up about bothersome side effects, such as nausea and vomiting. Ask about your options for managing or relieving the effects of treatment.

More information on nausea and vomiting is available at NCCN.org/patientguidelines and on the NCCN Patient Guides for Cancer app.

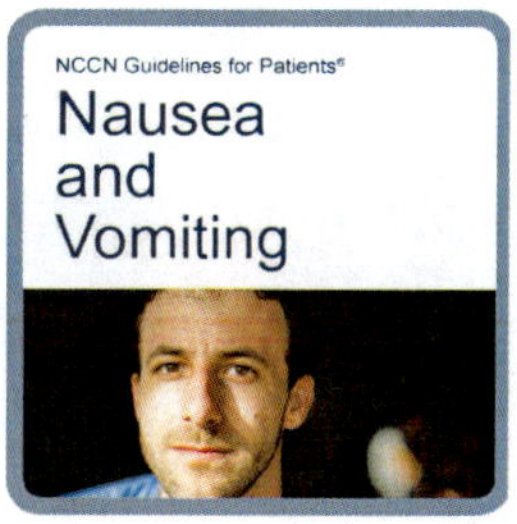

Medium-risk CHL

The following stages are generally considered to be intermediate (medium) risk:

- Bulky stage 1A and 2A cancers
- Some stage 1B, 2B, and 3A cancers

Preferred treatment options

If a clinical trial is not available or otherwise not an option, chemotherapy with one of the below regimens is preferred. The medicines included in these regimens are shown in **Guide 1** on page 32.

ABVE-PC

This option involves 4 cycles of ABVE-PC chemotherapy. After the first 2 cycles, you will have a PET scan to see how well treatment worked. The cancer will be designated as being either fast or slow to respond. Two more cycles of ABVE-PC will follow.

If the cancer was slow to respond to the first 2 cycles, or if cancer remains after 4 cycles, radiation therapy is recommended when chemotherapy is over.

OEPA and COPDAC

This option involves a total of 4 cycles of chemotherapy. After 2 cycles of OEPA, you will have a PET scan to see how well treatment worked. The cancer will be designated as being either fast or slow to respond. Two cycles of COPDAC chemotherapy will follow.

If the cancer was slow to respond to the first 2 cycles of chemotherapy, treating all original areas of cancer with radiation therapy is recommended after chemotherapy.

> “
>
> My advice is to allow patience and time to recuperate from Hodgkin lymphoma, for both patients and their parents/caregivers.
>
> - Hodgkin lymphoma survivor

Other recommended options

In some cases, regimens usually used for adults with Hodgkin lymphoma may be considered. Such regimens include ABVD and BEACOPP. These are often more toxic than the regimens usually used for young people with CHL.

High-risk CHL

The following stages are generally considered to be high risk:

- Some stage 2B and 3A cancers
- All stage 3B and stage 4 cancers

Preferred treatment options

If a clinical trial is not available or otherwise not an option, chemotherapy with one of the below regimens is preferred. The medicines included in these regimens are shown in **Guide 1** on the next page.

Bv-AVE-PC

This option involves 5 cycles of Bv-AVE-PC chemotherapy. After the first 2 cycles, you will have a PET scan to see how well treatment worked. The cancer will be designated as being either fast or slow to respond. Three more cycles of Bv-AVE-PC will follow.

When chemotherapy is over, any enlarged lymph nodes in the area between the lungs (called the mediastinum) will be treated with radiation therapy. If the cancer was slow to respond to the first 2 cycles of chemotherapy, the areas that were slow to improve—or did not improve—will also be treated with radiation.

OEPA and COPDAC

This option involves a total of 6 cycles of chemotherapy. After 2 cycles of OEPA, you will have a PET scan to see how well treatment worked. The cancer will be designated as being either fast or slow to respond. Four cycles of COPDAC chemotherapy will follow.

If the cancer was slow to respond to the first 2 cycles of chemotherapy, treating all original areas of cancer with radiation therapy is recommended.

Other recommended options

AEPA and CAPDAC

This option involves a total of 6 cycles of chemotherapy. After 2 cycles of AEPA, you will have a PET scan to see how well treatment worked. The cancer will be designated as being either fast or slow to respond. Four cycles of CAPDAC chemotherapy will follow. If the cancer was slow to respond to the first 2 cycles of chemotherapy, treating the areas that were slow to respond with radiation therapy is recommended after chemotherapy.

Less commonly used

The following chemotherapy regimens are used less often. They may be helpful in certain circumstances.

ABVE-PC

This option involves a total of 5 cycles of ABVE-PC chemotherapy. After the first 2 cycles, you will have a PET scan to see how well treatment worked. The cancer will be designated as being either fast or slow to respond. Three more cycles of ABVE-PC will follow.

When chemotherapy is over, any enlarged lymph nodes in the area between the lungs (called the mediastinum) will be treated with radiation therapy (ISRT). If the cancer was slow to respond to the first 2 cycles of chemotherapy, the areas that were slow to improve—or did not improve—will also be treated with radiation.

Adult regimens

In some cases, regimens usually used for adults with Hodgkin lymphoma may be considered. Such regimens include BEACOPP and ABVD. These are often more toxic than regimens recommended for young people with CHL.

Guide 1
Initial systemic therapy for classic Hodgkin lymphoma

Note: The regimens below may change as new information on the treatment of CHL becomes available.

OEPA	• Vincristine • Etoposide • Prednisone • Doxorubicin
AVPC (for the mixed cellularity type of CHL)	• Doxorubicin • Vincristine • Prednisone • Cyclophosphamide
ABVE-PC	• Doxorubicin • Bleomycin • Vincristine • Etoposide • Prednisone • Cyclophosphamide
Bv-AVE-PC (for high-risk disease)	• Brentuximab vedotin • Doxorubicin • Vincristine • Etoposide • Prednisone • Cyclophosphamide
COPDAC	• Cyclophosphamide • Vincristine • Prednisone • Dacarbazine
CAPDAC	• Cyclophosphamide • Brentuximab vedotin • Prednisone • Dacarbazine

When treatment is over

Hodgkin lymphoma and its treatment can cause serious health problems many years later. It is important to maintain a relationship with an oncologist who understands the health risks faced by Hodgkin lymphoma survivors. The recommended follow-up care after treatment is explained below.

Physical exams

Physical exams are an important part of follow-up care. They are given more often in the years right after treatment, and then spaced farther apart in later years.

First 1 to 2 years: Every 3 to 4 months

Until year 3: Every 6 to 12 months

Years 4 and 5: Once per year

Blood tests

There isn't a schedule for blood tests in the first few years after treatment. Your doctor may order bloodwork at the time of your physical exams, or only if relapse is suspected.

Recommended tests include a complete blood count (CBC), chemistry profile, and either erythrocyte sedimentation rate (ESR) or C-reactive protein (CRP).

If you had radiation therapy to the neck, a thyroid-stimulating hormone (TSH) test is recommended at least once a year.

Heart and lung tests

You may have lung function tests after treatment. Your doctor will consider this testing if chemotherapy included the drug bleomycin, or if the lungs were treated with radiation.

Good to know

There isn't a "one-size-fits-all" care plan that all Hodgkin lymphoma survivors should follow after treatment. The types of follow-up tests you should have—and how often you should have them—should be based on your specific cancer circumstances. This includes:

- ✓ Your age
- ✓ The cancer stage when you were diagnosed
- ✓ Your social habits
- ✓ Your treatment history

Your doctor may order an echocardiogram (heart ultrasound) when treatment is over. The goal is to get a baseline (starting) measurement of your heart health. The testing may then be repeated according to your risk of heart problems.

Imaging tests

There isn't a schedule for imaging after treatment. Your doctor will order imaging if you develop symptoms or if there are other possible signs of relapse, but no routine imaging is needed. If relapse is suspected, you may have a chest x-ray, CT with contrast, or MRI of all original areas of cancer.

If your most recent FDG-PET scan was a Deauville score of 3, 4, or 5, either an FDG-

PET/CT or PET/MRI scan is recommended when all treatment (including radiation therapy) is over. This is to make sure that no cancer can be detected. But having FDG-PET scans on a regular basis to monitor for the return of Hodgkin lymphoma is **not** recommended.

Vaccines

Everyone should continue to get the influenza vaccine (the "flu shot") every year, and other vaccines as needed. If the spleen was treated with radiation therapy, certain vaccines are recommended after treatment. These include the vaccines for pneumonia, meningitis, and Haemophilus influenzae type B ("Hib" or "H-flu"). Continue to let your doctors and imaging technologists know if you have had a COVID-19 vaccine prior to any imaging.

Survivorship

Side effects of Hodgkin lymphoma and its treatment can start years after treatment. These are called "late" side effects. The most serious late effects that Hodgkin survivors experience are described below.

Second cancers

Anyone who has had Hodgkin lymphoma is at risk of getting other types of cancer. This is especially true if radiation therapy was used as part of initial treatment. These "secondary cancers" often occur more than 10 years after treatment for Hodgkin lymphoma.

Thyroid cancer and breast cancer are the most common secondary cancers diagnosed in Hodgkin lymphoma survivors. Skin cancers can also occur in areas treated with radiation.

Survivorship counseling

Hodgkin lymphoma survivors are encouraged to undergo counseling on survivorship, including long-term treatment effects, preventing new cancers, and healthy behaviors. Ask your doctor about survivorship clinics near you.

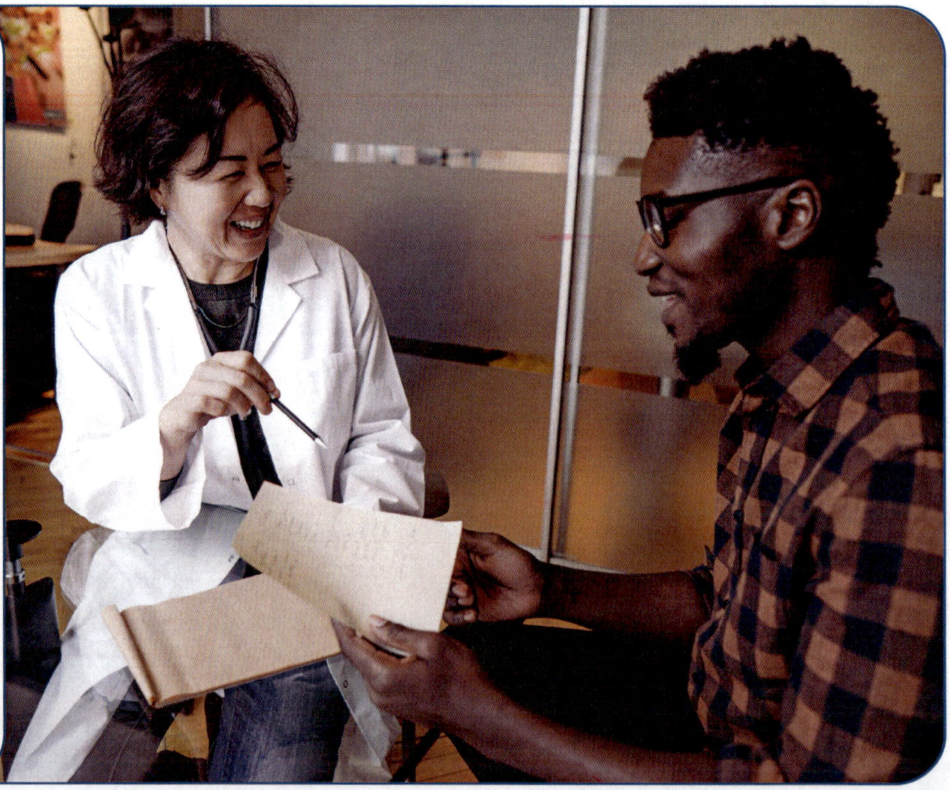

Thyroid problems

The thyroid is a small, butterfly-shaped gland in the front of the neck. About half of Hodgkin lymphoma survivors who had radiation therapy to the neck or upper chest have thyroid problems later in life. The most common problem is hypothyroidism, in which the thyroid gland doesn't make enough thyroid hormone.

Weight gain, constipation, dry skin, and sensitivity to cold temperatures are symptoms of an underactive thyroid. Your doctor should do a careful thyroid examination during your annual physical exam.

Thyroid function tests should also be done at least once a year to rule out hypothyroidism, especially in people who had radiation therapy to the neck.

Heart disease

Hodgkin lymphoma survivors have a higher long-term risk of diseases that affect the heart or blood vessels. This is called heart disease or cardiovascular disease. Symptoms of heart disease can start at any age, but damage to the heart or blood vessels is usually found more than 5 to 10 years after finishing treatment.

The biggest risk factors for developing heart disease in Hodgkin lymphoma survivors are:

- Treatment with radiation therapy to the area between the lungs
- Treatment with chemotherapy medicines called anthracyclines

Doxorubicin is an anthracycline used in some chemotherapy regimens used to treat Hodgkin lymphoma in young people, including OEPA.

Everyone treated for Hodgkin lymphoma should have their blood pressure checked at least once a year, even if there are no symptoms of heart disease.

Survivorship counseling

Ask your doctor about:

- What to expect now that treatment is over
- Fertility and family planning issues
- Leading a healthy lifestyle after cancer treatment
- The risk of other cancers, especially thyroid and breast cancer, and steps to help prevent them
- Taking care of your mental and emotional health
- Survivorship support groups and/or clinics

For more information on cancer survivorship, the following are available at NCCN.org/patientguidelines and on the NCCN Patient Guides for Cancer app:

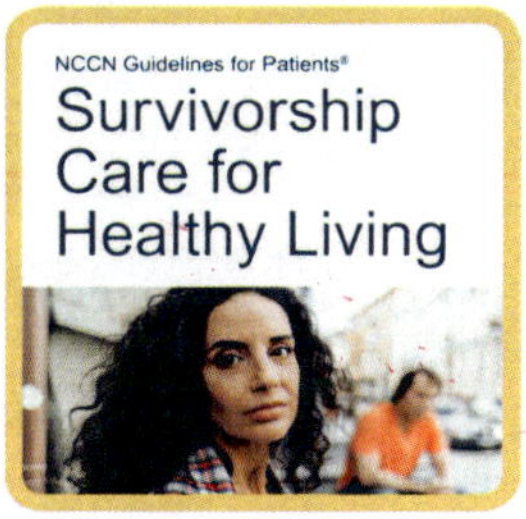

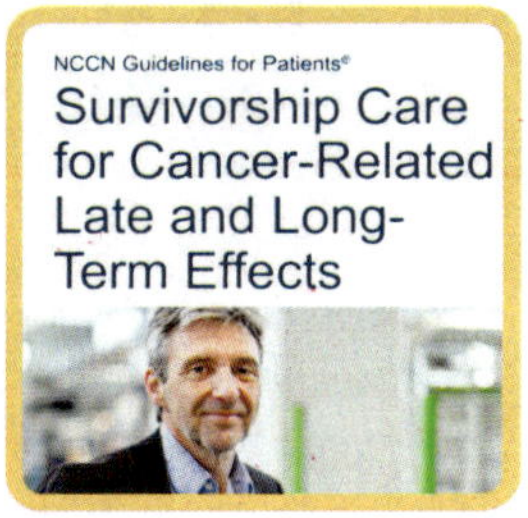

These resources address:

- Anxiety, depression, and distress
- Fatigue
- Pain
- Sexual problems
- Sleep problems
- Healthy lifestyles
- Work, insurance, and disability

Relapse

Most young people with Hodgkin lymphoma stay cancer-free after treatment. But about 1 in 10 will experience a relapse, or the return of cancer.

If a relapse is suspected, a biopsy is needed to confirm areas of suspected cancer before starting treatment. This allows your doctor to see what is in the tumor and plan treatment accordingly. If confirmed, enrollment in a clinical trial for treatment is strongly encouraged. Your doctor should also refer you to a specialized cancer center or consult closely with a center with expertise in Hodgkin lymphoma.

If a clinical trial is not available, relapsed CHL is usually treated with chemotherapy first. Immunotherapy may also be used, either by itself or with chemotherapy. When used to treat relapse, systemic therapy is called **re-induction therapy**. Currently recommended regimens are listed in **Guide 2**.

Guide 2
Systemic therapy for relapsed Hodgkin lymphoma

The regimens listed below may change as new information on treating relapsed CHL becomes available.

Options to try first for re-induction (in alphabetical order)	• Brentuximab vedotin + bendamustine, gemcitabine, or nivolumab • DHAP (dexamethasone + cytarabine + cisplatin) • GV (gemcitabine + vinorelbine) • IGEV (ifosfamide + gemcitabine + vinorelbine) • IV (ifosfamide + vinorelbine)
Options to try next	**Chemotherapy**: • Re-induction regimens listed above that weren't tried • Bortezomib + ifosfamide + vinorelbine • EPIC (etoposide + prednisolone + ifosfamide + cisplatin) • GDP (gemcitabine + dexamethasone + cisplatin) • ICE (ifosfamide + carboplatin + etoposide) **Immunotherapy:** • Nivolumab (Opdivo) or pembrolizumab (Keytruda)
Maintenance (after stem cell transplant)	Brentuximab vedotin (for some people with high-risk disease)

The goal is to achieve a complete response to re-induction therapy. This means that no cancer can be detected. Chemotherapy with more than one re-induction regimen may be needed to get a complete response. If achieved, a stem cell transplant is usually recommended next for those that relapse within the first year after the end of treatment. More information on this procedure is provided below. Radiation therapy may follow the transplant.

For some very-low-risk cases of relapse, it may be possible to avoid a stem cell transplant. Treatment with re-induction therapy and radiation therapy may be given instead. Avoiding a stem cell transplant may be possible if:

- The cancer stage at diagnosis was **not** 3B or 4B
- You have not received any radiation therapy
- You were cancer-free for at least a year after initial treatment
- Cancer has not spread outside any lymph nodes
- You do not have B symptoms (fevers, night sweats, weight loss).

After re-induction therapy and either stem cell transplant and/or radiation therapy, your doctor will order an FDG-PET scan to check the results. If no cancer can be seen, observation will start. You will have a follow-up exam shortly thereafter. If the FDG-PET scan shows areas of cancer, more systemic therapy is recommended. Options to try next are listed in **Guide 2**.

Immunotherapy

If the cancer returns after treatment with at least 2 different chemotherapy regimens, and immunotherapy has not yet been used, treatment with an immune checkpoint inhibitor should be strongly considered.

Examples include nivolumab (Opdivo) and pembrolizumab (Keytruda). Checkpoint inhibitors work by increasing the activity of the immune system. This improves the body's ability to find and destroy cancer cells.

If immunotherapy is planned, more information on the side effects of checkpoint inhibitors is available at NCCN.org/patientguidelines and on the NCCN Patient Guides for Cancer app.

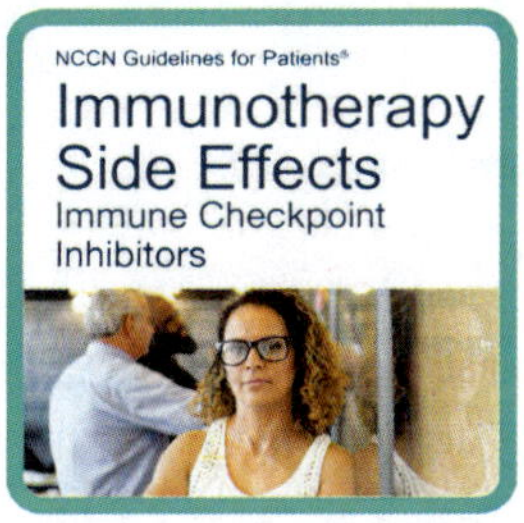

High-dose chemotherapy with stem cell rescue

High-dose chemotherapy may be used to treat relapsed or refractory Hodgkin lymphoma. Refractory means that the cancer was not cured with initial treatment. Relapsed means that the cancer returned after successful treatment.

Such high doses of chemotherapy can damage or destroy hematopoietic (blood-forming) stem cells, which are found in the bone marrow.

When damaged, they may not form the blood cells needed by the body. To protect your blood-forming stem cells from high-dose chemotherapy, some stem cells are removed from your blood weeks or months before this treatment is started. They are stored in a lab.

After the high-dose chemotherapy regimen has been completed, your bone marrow will be "rescued" by giving back your healthy stem cells. The transplanted stem cells will form new red blood cells, white blood cells, and platelets. This will restore your body's ability to protect itself from infection. It will also helps prevent bleeding.

A number of names are used to refer to this procedure, including:

- High-dose therapy with autologous stem cell rescue (HDT/ASCR)
- Autologous stem cell transplant
- Hematopoietic cell transplant (HCT)

The stem cell rescue process

The first step is to increase the number of stem cells in the blood. This is known as mobilization. Medicines are used to cause stem cells to move from the bone marrow into the blood. When your doctor determines that your stem cell count is high enough, the next step is collection.

A process called apheresis is used to collect the stem cells from blood. Your blood will be removed from a large vein, most likely in your arm. It will flow through a tube and into a machine that removes stem cells. The rest of your blood will be returned to you in your other arm. Apheresis typically takes around 4 to 6 hours and does not require anesthesia. It

Stem cell rescue

High-dose chemotherapy may be used to treat relapsed or refractory cancer. To protect blood-forming stem cells found in bone marrow, some are removed from your blood weeks or months beforehand. When high-dose chemotherapy is over, your bone marrow is "rescued" by giving back your healthy stem cells.

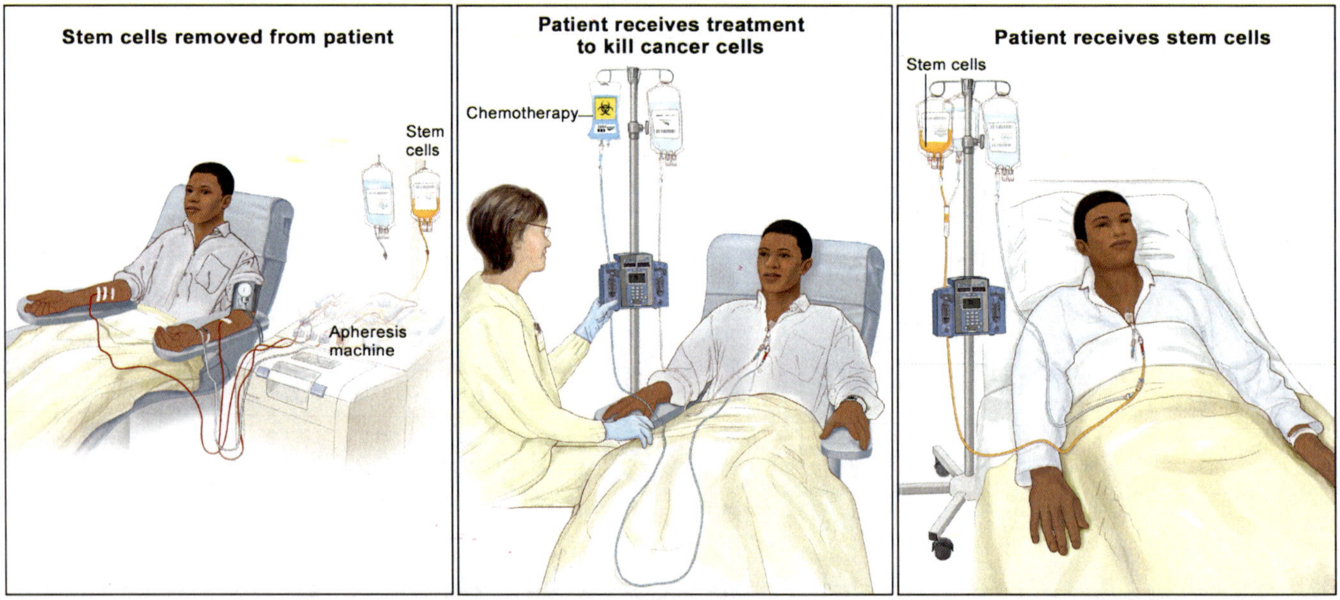

may take 2 or more sessions to obtain enough stem cells. During the procedure, you may have lightheadedness, chills, numbness around the lips, and cramping in the hands. After apheresis, the collected ("harvested") cells are frozen and stored.

When high-dose chemotherapy is complete, your harvested stem cells will be put back into your body using a transfusion. A transfusion is a slow injection of blood products through a central line into a large vein. A central line (or central venous catheter) is a thin tube that is inserted into your skin through one incision (cut), then into your vein through a second cut. Local or general anesthesia will be used, depending on the circumstances. Sometimes a percutaneously inserted central catheter (PICC) line can be used for the transplant. This is a thin catheter that is inserted into a blood vessel in your arm, and then advanced to a larger blood vessel that leads to the heart. This procedure usually requires just local anesthesia.

The transplanted stem cells travel to your bone marrow where they grow and form new, healthy blood cells. This is called engraftment and usually takes about 2 to 4 weeks. Until engraftment is fully achieved, your immune system will not be able to fight infections very well. You will need to stay in a very clean room at the hospital with a special air filtration system.

You may be given an antibiotic to prevent or treat infection. If your platelet count is low, you may also be given platelet infusions to prevent bleeding. Red blood cell transfusions may be given if your hemoglobin is low (anemia). While waiting for the cells to engraft, you will likely feel tired and weak.

Key points

Treatment

- Chemotherapy is the most effective treatment for Hodgkin lymphoma.
- Options for chemotherapy are based on the risk level of the cancer.
- Radiation therapy may be given after chemotherapy.
- Regardless of risk level, seeking treatment within a clinical trial is encouraged when possible.

When treatment is over

- Hodgkin lymphoma and its treatment can cause breast, thyroid, and other cancers many years later.
- Thyroid problems and heart disease are other possible late effects.
- Physical exams are recommended on a regular basis during the first 5 years after treatment.
- Other testing is generally ordered as needed if relapse is suspected.

Relapse

- If a clinical trial is not an option, relapsed CHL is usually treated with chemotherapy first. This is called re-induction therapy.
- If re-induction therapy works very well, high-dose chemotherapy with stem cell rescue is often the next step. Sometimes radiation therapy is an option instead.
- If cancer returns after several rounds of chemotherapy, immunotherapy with a checkpoint inhibitor should be considered.

5

Treatment for nodular lymphocyte-predominant Hodgkin lymphoma (NLPHL)

NLPHL is a rare type of Hodgkin lymphoma. It is usually very small and treatable when found. But its treatment can cause late side effects. Long-term follow-up is essential.

Unlike classic Hodgkin lymphoma (CHL), most people with NLPHL have had a lymph node growing for several (more than 2) years. They also don't usually have fevers, night sweats, or weight loss. In young people, NLPHL also tends to be found at an earlier age than CHL and more often in those assigned male sex at birth.

The chemotherapy regimens used for early-stage CHL are also used for NLPHL. These regimens work well but often overtreat the disease. The chemotherapy and possibly radiation therapy used can cause side effects years later, including other cancers. NLPHL can also transform into a fast-growing type of non-Hodgkin lymphoma called diffuse large B-cell lymphoma.

An antibody therapy called rituximab (Rituxan) is sometimes added to chemotherapy to treat NLPHL. Rituximab targets and attaches to a protein found on the surface of NLPHL cells (and some healthy blood cells). This helps the immune system find and attack the cancer cells.

Early-stage NLPHL

Most people have early-stage NLPHL at the time of diagnosis. Early-stage NLPHL includes stages 1A and 2A. Most of these tumors are small (not bulky). The following information applies to non-bulky stage 1A or 2A NLPHL. The letter A after the stage means that the cancer is not causing "B" symptoms.

Surgery to remove the cancer is recommended. A positron emission tomography/computed tomography (PET/CT) scan is done afterward to learn if all of the cancer was removed. Further treatment, if needed, depends on the results of surgery.

Complete resection

If the results of surgery are very good, it is called complete resection. After complete resection, there are 2 **preferred** options for next steps. The first is enrolling in an ongoing clinical trial. The other is observation.

Observation involves monitoring the original cancer site with imaging. An ultrasound is recommended every 3 to 4 months for the first 2 years after surgery. Two out of 3 people with NLPHL will be cured with surgery alone.

While observation alone is preferred for those with a complete resection, chemotherapy is also an option. If chemotherapy is planned, 3 cycles of the CVbP regimen is recommended. Rituximab may be added. The medicines included in the CVbP regimen are listed in **Guide 3** on the next page.

For those above 18 years of age, regimens normally used for adults with Hodgkin lymphoma may be considered instead of CVbP.

Incomplete resection

Sometimes the cancer cannot be fully removed during surgery. This is called incomplete resection. The following information applies to those with non-bulky stage 1A or 2A cancer that was incompletely resected.

There are 2 **preferred** options. The first is enrolling in an ongoing trial. If a clinical trial is not available or otherwise not an option, chemotherapy is recommended. Three cycles of one of the below regimens is preferred.

- AVPC
- CVbP (rituximab may be added)

The medicines included in these regimens are listed in **Guide 3**.

If the cancer responds well to chemotherapy, no further treatment is needed. Follow-up care will begin.

If cancer remains after 3 cycles of chemotherapy, radiation therapy is recommended. Or you may be referred to a specialty center for further treatment.

Other recommended options

Another recommended option is 2 cycles of OEPA chemotherapy. If cancer remains after 2 cycles, radiation therapy is recommended. Or you may be referred to a specialty center for further treatment.

For patients above 18 years of age, regimens normally used for adults with Hodgkin lymphoma may also be considered.

Guide 3
Systemic therapy for NLPHL

CVbP	• Cyclophosphamide • Vinblastine • Prednisolone • Maybe also rituximab
AVPC	• Doxorubicin • Vincristine • Prednisone • Cyclophosphamide
OEPA	• Vincristine • Etoposide • Prednisone • Doxorubicin

Advanced NLPHL

The stages listed below are considered advanced.

- Bulky stage 1A and 2A
- Stage 1B and 2B
- Stage 3
- Stage 4

Advanced-stage NLPHL is very rare in young people. If advanced disease is suspected, a double-check of the diagnosis is recommended. An expert pathologist should review the original tissue samples to confirm that the cancer is NLPHL.

If confirmed, treatment at a specialty cancer center is recommended when possible. Due to a lack of data, advanced NLPHL is often treated similarly to classic Hodgkin lymphoma.

Follow-up care

The same follow-up care that is recommended for classic Hodgkin lymphoma is also recommended for NLPHL. See page 33 for more information.

Key points

- NLPHL is a rare type of Hodgkin lymphoma. It is usually small and treatable when found.

Early-stage NLPHL

- Surgery is the recommended first treatment for early-stage NLPHL. If the results are very good, it is called complete resection.
- After complete resection, observation or a clinical trial are preferred options. CVbP chemotherapy is also a recommended option.
- After incomplete resection, preferred options are a clinical trial and either AVPC or CVbP chemotherapy. OEPA chemotherapy is also a recommended option.
- If cancer remains after chemotherapy with AVPC, CVbP, or OEPA, radiation therapy is recommended.

Advanced NLPHL

- Advanced NLPHL is very rare in young people. The diagnosis should be confirmed.
- Treatment at a specialty cancer center is recommended for advanced NLPHL when possible.
- Due to a lack of data, advanced NLPHL is often treated much like classic Hodgkin lymphoma.

Follow-up care

- Treatment for NLPHL can cause side effects years afterward.
- Long-term follow-up is essential.

6

Making treatment decisions

It's important to be comfortable with the cancer treatment you choose. This choice starts with having an open and honest conversation with your care team.

It's your choice

In shared decision-making, you and your doctors share information, discuss the options, and agree on a treatment plan. It starts with an open and honest conversation between you and your doctor.

Treatment decisions are very personal. What is important to you may not be important to someone else.

Some things that may play a role in your decision-making:

- What you want and how that might differ from what others want
- Your religious and spiritual beliefs
- Your feelings about certain treatments
- Your feelings about pain or side effects
- Cost of treatment, travel to treatment centers, and time away from school or work
- Quality of life and length of life
- How active you are and the activities that are important to you

Think about what you want from treatment. Discuss openly the risks and benefits of specific treatments and procedures. Weigh options and share concerns with your doctor.

If you take the time to build a relationship with your doctor, it will help you feel supported when considering options and making treatment decisions.

Second opinion

It is normal to want to start treatment as soon as possible. While cancer can't be ignored, there is time to have another doctor review your test results and suggest a treatment plan. This is called getting a second opinion, and it's a normal part of cancer care. It will not upset your treatment team. Even doctors get second opinions!

Things you can do to prepare:

- Check with your insurance company about its rules on second opinions. There may be out-of-pocket costs to see doctors who are not part of your insurance plan.
- Make plans to have copies of all your records sent to the doctor you will see for your second opinion.

Support groups

Many people diagnosed with cancer find support groups to be helpful. Support groups often include people at different stages of treatment. Some people may be newly diagnosed, while others may be finished with treatment. If your hospital or community doesn't have support groups for people with cancer, check out the websites listed in this book.

Questions to ask

Possible questions to ask your doctors are listed on the following pages. Feel free to use these questions or come up with your own. Be clear about your goals for treatment and find out what to expect from treatment.

Questions about cancer testing

1. What type of biopsy did I (or will I) have?
2. What is the cancer stage?
3. What other tests will I have?
4. Will my insurance pay for all of the recommended tests?
5. How can I get a copy of the pathology report and other test results?
6. Is there an online portal with my test results?

Questions about treatment options

1. What are my treatment options? Do they include clinical trials?
2. Are you suggesting options other than what NCCN recommends? If yes, why?
3. What are the risks and benefits of joining a clinical trial?
4. How do I find clinical trials that I can participate in?
5. How do my age, sex, overall health, and other factors affect my options?
6. What if I am pregnant, or planning to become pregnant?
7. Does any option offer a cure or long-term cancer control?
8. How do I get a second opinion?
9. How long do I have to decide about treatment?

Questions about classic Hodgkin lymphoma (CHL)

1. What is the cancer subtype (nodular sclerosis, mixed cellularity, lymphocyte-rich, or lymphocyte-depleted)?
2. What is the cancer stage?
3. Which chemotherapy regimen do you recommend for me?
4. Is it different than what NCCN recommends? If yes, why?
5. What are the most common side effects of the chemotherapy regimen you are recommending?
6. How long will chemotherapy last?
7. Will you stop or change regimens if there are serious side effects?
8. Will I need radiation therapy after chemotherapy?
9. If so, how long will radiation therapy last? Which areas will be treated?
10. What are the chances of the cancer worsening or returning?

Questions about nodular lymphocyte-predominant Hodgkin lymphoma (NLPHL)

1. What stage is the cancer?
2. Is it bulky?
3. Am I a candidate for surgery first?
4. Can you provide more information on what surgery will involve?
5. Is complete resection common?
6. How do you know if the cancer has started to transform?
7. What are the chances of the cancer worsening or returning?

Questions about your care team

1. What is your experience treating childhood Hodgkin lymphoma?
2. Does this hospital or cancer center offer the best treatment for me?
3. How many people like me (of the same age, gender, race) have you treated?
4. Will you be consulting with experts to discuss my care? Whom will you consult?
5. Whom should I contact with questions or concerns if the office is closed?
6. What supportive care and services are available to me and my caregivers?

Resources

Be The Match
BeTheMatch.org/one-on-one

Cancer Hope Network
cancerhopenetwork.org

Lymphoma Research Foundation
lymphoma.org/understanding-lymphoma/aboutlymphoma/hl

The Leukemia & Lymphoma Society (LLS)
LLS.org/PatientSupport

Triage Cancer
triagecancer.org

We want your feedback!

Our goal is to provide helpful and easy-to-understand information on cancer.

Take our survey to let us know what we got right and what we could do better.

NCCN.org/patients/feedback

Words to know

abdomen
The area of the body between the chest and pelvis. Contains the pancreas, stomach, bowel, liver, gallbladder, and other organs.

B symptoms
High fevers, heavy night sweats, and fast weight loss without dieting caused by Hodgkin lymphoma.

bone marrow
Soft, sponge-like tissue in the center of most bones where blood cells are made.

cancer stage
A rating of the extent of cancer in the body.

chemotherapy
The use of anti-cancer medicines. A type of systemic therapy.

classic Hodgkin lymphoma (CHL)
The most common type of Hodgkin lymphoma. Subtypes include nodular sclerosis, mixed cellularity, lymphocyte-rich, and lymphocyte-depleted.

clinical trial
A type of research that studies how well investigational treatments work in people.

contrast
A substance put into the body to make clearer pictures during imaging tests.

Deauville scale
A rating by doctors of treatment response based on comparing the uptake of a radiotracer by cancer sites to 2 other sites.

diaphragm
The thin muscle below the lungs and heart that helps a person to breathe.

echocardiogram
An ultrasound of the heart. Recommended if chemotherapy containing an anthracycline is planned.

erythrocyte sedimentation rate (ESR)
A blood test that measures how quickly red blood cells settle at the bottom of a test tube containing a blood sample.

excisional biopsy
A preferred type of biopsy for diagnosing childhood Hodgkin lymphoma. Involves removing entire lymph nodes to test for cancer cells.

incisional biopsy
A preferred type of biopsy for diagnosing childhood Hodgkin lymphoma. Involves removing a small amount of lymph node tissue through a cut in the skin.

involved-site radiation therapy (ISRT)
A type of external radiation therapy often used to treat Hodgkin lymphoma. Radiation is delivered to the lymph nodes in which the cancer started and nearby areas of cancer.

lung function test
A test used to measure how well the lungs work. Also called pulmonary function test.

lymph
A clear fluid containing white blood cells called lymphocytes.

lymphatic system
The tissues and organs that produce, store, and carry white blood cells that fight infections and other diseases. Part of the immune system.

lymph node
Small groups of disease-fighting cells located throughout the body.

lymphocyte
A type of immune cell that is made in the bone marrow and is found in the blood and in lymph tissue.

mediastinum
The area of the chest between the lungs.

nodular lymphocyte-predominant Hodgkin lymphoma (NLPHL)
A rare form of Hodgkin lymphoma that can transform into a fast-growing type of non-Hodgkin lymphoma.

positron emission tomography (PET) scan
A test that uses a small amount of radioactive glucose (sugar) and a scanner to see where cancer may still exist in the body.

spleen
An organ in the lymphatic system that helps protect the body from disease. It is located on the left side of the abdomen near the stomach.

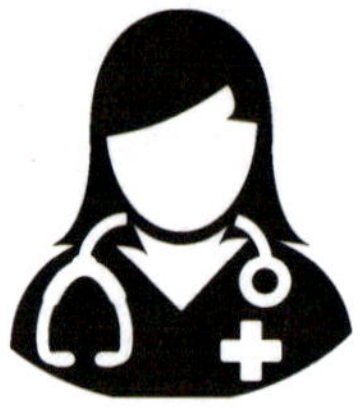

Hodgkin lymphoma is curable because of clinical trials. Young people with this uncommon cancer are strongly encouraged to enroll in a clinical trial for treatment. More information on clinical trials is provided in the first chapter of this guide.

NCCN Contributors

This patient guide is based on the NCCN Clinical Practice Guidelines in Oncology (NCCN Guidelines®) for Pediatric Hodgkin Lymphoma, Version 2.2023. It was adapted, reviewed, and published with help from the following people:

Dorothy A. Shead, MS
Senior Director
Patient Information Operations

Erin Vidic, MA
Senior Medical Writer, Patient Information

Laura Phillips
Graphic Artist

The NCCN Clinical Practice Guidelines in Oncology (NCCN Guidelines®) for Pediatric Hodgkin Lymphoma, Version 2.2023 were developed by the following NCCN Panel Members:

*Jamie E. Flerlage, MD, MS/Chair
St. Jude Children's Research Hospital/ The University of Tennessee Health Science Center

Susan M. Hiniker, MD/Vice Chair
Stanford Cancer Institute

Saro Armenian, DO, MPH
City of Hope National Medical Center

Jennifer Belsky, DO, MS
Indiana University Melvin and Bren Simon Comprehensive Cancer Center

*Adam J. Bobbey, MD
The Ohio State University Comprehensive Cancer Center - James Cancer Hospital and Solove Research Institute

Vivian Chang, MD
UCLA Jonsson Comprehensive Cancer Center

Stacy Cooper, MD
The Sidney Kimmel Comprehensive Cancer Center at Johns Hopkins

Don W. Coulter, MD
Fred & Pamela Buffett Cancer Center

Branko Cuglievan, MD
The University of Texas MD Anderson Cancer Center

*Kenneth DeSantes, MD
University of Wisconsin Carbone Cancer Center

Anusha Preethi Ganesan, MD, PhD
Rady Children's Hospital-San Diego/ UC San Diego Moores Cancer Center

Chelsee Greer, DO
UT Southwestern Simmons Comprehensive Cancer Center

Mallorie Heneghan, MD, MS
Huntsman Cancer Institute at the University of Utah

Bradford S. Hoppe, MD, MPH
Mayo Clinic Comprehensive Cancer Center

Leidy Isenalumhe, MD, MS
Moffitt Cancer Center

Kara Kelly, MD
Roswell Park Comprehensive Cancer Center

Leslie Kersun, MD, MSCE, MSEd
Children's Hospital of Philadelphia/ Abramson Cancer Center at the University of Pennsylvania

Adam J. Lamble, MD
Fred Hutchinson Cancer Center

Nicole A. Larrier, MD, MSc
Duke Cancer Institute

Sandra Luna-Fineman, MD
University of Colorado Cancer Center

*Jeffrey Magee, MD, PhD
Siteman Cancer Center at Barnes-Jewish Hospital and Washington University School of Medicine

Kwadwo Oduro, MD, PhD
Case Comprehensive Cancer Center/ University Hospitals Seidman Cancer Center and Cleveland Clinic Taussig Cancer Institute

Arun Ranjan Panigrahi, MD
UC Davis Comprehensive Cancer Center

Anita P. Price, MD
Memorial Sloan Kettering Cancer Center

Kenneth B. Roberts, MD
Yale Cancer Center/Smilow Cancer Hospital

Christine M. Smith, MD
Vanderbilt-Ingram Cancer Center

*Aliyah R. Sohani, MD
Mass General Cancer Center

*Emily Walling, MD, MPHS
University of Michigan Rogel Cancer Center

Jane N. Winter, MD
Robert H. Lurie Comprehensive Cancer Center of Northwestern University

Ana C. Xavier, MD
O'Neal Comprehensive Cancer Center at UAB

NCCN

Deborah Freedman-Cass, PhD
Senior Manager, Guidelines Processes

Megan Lyons, MS
Associate Scientist/Medical Writer

Katie Stehman, PA-C
Oncology Scientist/Medical Writer

* Reviewed this patient guide. For disclosures, visit NCCN.org/disclosures.

NCCN Cancer Centers

Abramson Cancer Center
at the University of Pennsylvania
Philadelphia, Pennsylvania
800.789.7366 • pennmedicine.org/cancer

Case Comprehensive Cancer Center/
University Hospitals Seidman Cancer Center and
Cleveland Clinic Taussig Cancer Institute
Cleveland, Ohio
UH Seidman Cancer Center
800.641.2422 • uhhospitals.org/services/cancer-services
CC Taussig Cancer Institute
866.223.8100 • my.clevelandclinic.org/departments/cancer
Case CCC
216.844.8797 • case.edu/cancer

City of Hope National Medical Center
Duarte, California
800.826.4673 • cityofhope.org

Dana-Farber/Brigham and Women's Cancer Center |
Mass General Cancer Center
Boston, Massachusetts
617.732.5500 • youhaveus.org
617.726.5130 • massgeneral.org/cancer-center

Duke Cancer Institute
Durham, North Carolina
888.275.3853 • dukecancerinstitute.org

Fox Chase Cancer Center
Philadelphia, Pennsylvania
888.369.2427 • foxchase.org

Fred & Pamela Buffett Cancer Center
Omaha, Nebraska
402.559.5600 • unmc.edu/cancercenter

Fred Hutchinson Cancer Center
Seattle, Washington
206.667.5000 • fredhutch.org

Huntsman Cancer Institute at the University of Utah
Salt Lake City, Utah
800.824.2073 • huntsmancancer.org

Indiana University Melvin and Bren Simon
Comprehensive Cancer Center
Indianapolis, Indiana
888.600.4822 • www.cancer.iu.edu

Mayo Clinic Comprehensive Cancer Center
Phoenix/Scottsdale, Arizona
Jacksonville, Florida
Rochester, Minnesota
480.301.8000 • Arizona
904.953.0853 • Florida
507.538.3270 • Minnesota
mayoclinic.org/cancercenter

Memorial Sloan Kettering Cancer Center
New York, New York
800.525.2225 • mskcc.org

Moffitt Cancer Center
Tampa, Florida
888.663.3488 • moffitt.org

O'Neal Comprehensive Cancer Center at UAB
Birmingham, Alabama
800.822.0933 • uab.edu/onealcancercenter

Robert H. Lurie Comprehensive Cancer Center
of Northwestern University
Chicago, Illinois
866.587.4322 • cancer.northwestern.edu

Roswell Park Comprehensive Cancer Center
Buffalo, New York
877.275.7724 • roswellpark.org

Siteman Cancer Center at Barnes-Jewish Hospital
and Washington University School of Medicine
St. Louis, Missouri
800.600.3606 • siteman.wustl.edu

St. Jude Children's Research Hospital/
The University of Tennessee Health Science Center
Memphis, Tennessee
866.278.5833 • stjude.org
901.448.5500 • uthsc.edu

Stanford Cancer Institute
Stanford, California
877.668.7535 • cancer.stanford.edu

The Ohio State University Comprehensive Cancer Center -
James Cancer Hospital and Solove Research Institute
Columbus, Ohio
800.293.5066 • cancer.osu.edu

The Sidney Kimmel Comprehensive
Cancer Center at Johns Hopkins
Baltimore, Maryland
410.955.8964
www.hopkinskimmelcancercenter.org

The UChicago Medicine Comprehensive Cancer Center
Chicago, Illinois
773.702.1000 • uchicagomedicine.org/cancer

The University of Texas MD Anderson Cancer Center
Houston, Texas
844.269.5922 • mdanderson.org

UC Davis Comprehensive Cancer Center
Sacramento, California
916.734.5959 • 800.770.9261
health.ucdavis.edu/cancer

UC San Diego Moores Cancer Center
La Jolla, California
858.822.6100 • cancer.ucsd.edu

UCLA Jonsson Comprehensive Cancer Center
Los Angeles, California
310.825.5268 • cancer.ucla.edu

UCSF Helen Diller Family
Comprehensive Cancer Center
San Francisco, California
800.689.8273 • cancer.ucsf.edu

University of Colorado Cancer Center
Aurora, Colorado
720.848.0300 • coloradocancercenter.org

University of Michigan Rogel Cancer Center
Ann Arbor, Michigan
800.865.1125 • rogelcancercenter.org

University of Wisconsin Carbone Cancer Center
Madison, Wisconsin
608.265.1700 • uwhealth.org/cancer

UT Southwestern Simmons
Comprehensive Cancer Center
Dallas, Texas
214.648.3111 • utsouthwestern.edu/simmons

Vanderbilt-Ingram Cancer Center
Nashville, Tennessee
877.936.8422 • vicc.org

Yale Cancer Center/Smilow Cancer Hospital
New Haven, Connecticut
855.4.SMILOW • yalecancercenter.org

Index